The Street Knowledge Family Guide
of
Drug Prevention
"Healthier Living Series"

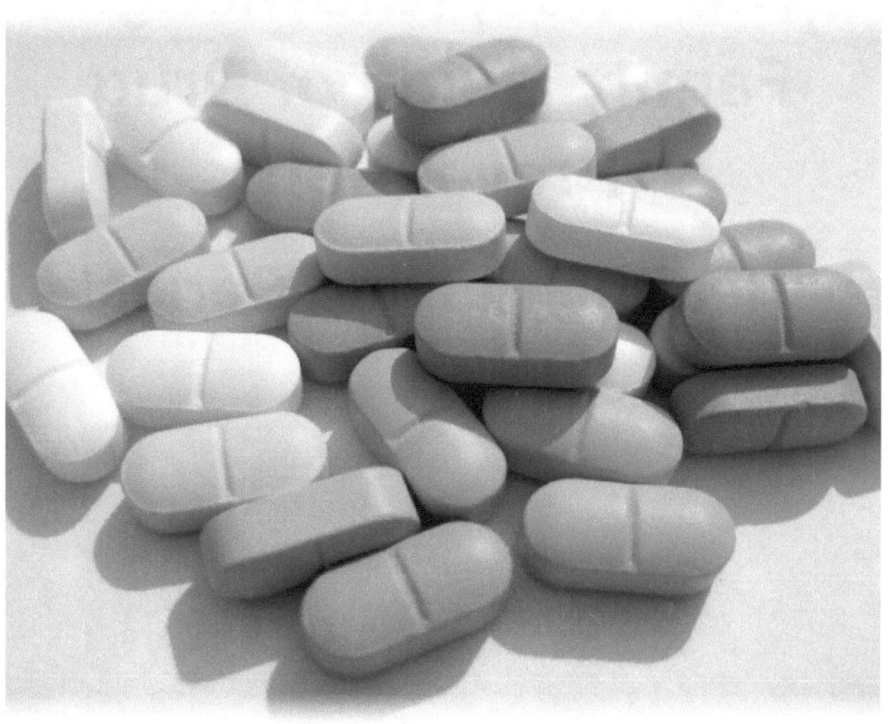

The Street Knowledge Family Guide of Drug Prevention

"Healthier Living Series"

The Street Knowledge Family Guide of Drug Prevention

"Healthier Living Series"

Franklin Gillette

Printed by Lulu Press

Copyright

The Street Knowledge Family Guide of Drug Prevention
"Healthier Living Series"
 by Franklin Gillette

First Edition

More from This Author Franklin

- **Compatibility: Code of Harmony**
  for Love and Unity
  "Happier Relationship Series"
- **Automatic Natural Weight Loss system**
  "Healthier Living Series"
- **How to Protect Yourself, Family, Property and**
  Valuables from Crime in
  Public or at Home
  "Household Solutions Series"
- **How to Make Extra Money**
  at Home Right now
  "Greater Wealth Series"

Table of Contents

INTRODUCTION

Parents! Help your child say NO to drugs! Together you must agree to avoid Marijuana, Crank, Ice, Crack, AIDS, LSD, Jail, PCP, and Gangs!

If you're a parent or young adult, you know there's a drug problem in this country. Whether its alcohol, the most abused drug of all, or crack cocaine, one of the most psychologically addictive drugs, the problem affects us all.

Over 70 million people in U.S. households have used illegal drugs. A large percentage of crime can be directly linked to the drug trade. Thefts, burglaries, and robberies (and murders committed during the commission of these crimes) are committed for the sole purpose of financing drug habits. Drug use harms many, many more people than just the drug user!

This book is designed to help families deal with one of America's biggest problems... drug abuse. No technical jargon - No boring lecture. Just the facts in street language. Learn how to identify the various drugs, find out how they're used, the signs of their use, the consequence of their use, and more! Whether its alcohol, the most abused of all drugs, or crack, one of the most dangerous and psychologically addictive drugs, you'll get the inside information you and your child need.

Chapter 1

Possible Signs of Drug Use

If you're a parent or young adult, you know there's a drug problem on this planet. Whether it's alcohol; the most abused drug, or crack cocaine; one of the most psychologically addictive and dangerous drugs, the problem affects us all.

Federal studies show that over 70 million people in U.S. households have used illegal drugs! Drugs are responsible for a great number of the crimes committed today! Thefts, burglaries, robberies and murders a recommitted for the sole purpose of financing drug habits!

This book is presented only as a source of general information. Nothing in this report is to be considered as legal or medical advice! Consult with legal and medical professionals for the best advice on topics covered in this report. Parents are encouraged to add their own views and suggestions to each topic. Lastly, this book is not intended to replace a parent's instructions to their children.

Alcohol is the most abused of all drugs! It is believed that almost three quarters of the U.S. population uses alcohol to some extent. Alcohol enters the bloodstream quickly and affects the judgment and behavior of the user. It affects coordination and response time. Thousands of teenagers are killed each year in alcohol-related traffic accidents!

Marijuana is the most abused of all the illegal drugs. It is normally smoked in hand-rolled cigarettes, pipes, and other suitable devices. It is also ingested by mixing in food and drink. Marijuana is a mind-altering drug that causes a state of intoxication. It can affect thinking and judgment and can cause anxiety attacks. Marijuana use can cause tissue damage, panic attacks, bronchitis, and changes in male hormones. It has more cancer causing chemicals than tobacco!

Marijuana is made from the leaves and flowering tops of the cannabis sativa plant, which are harvested and dried. The mind-altering component of Marijuana is called THC, for short. The higher the THC content, the more potent the Marijuana. Hashish is a resin that is extracted from the marijuana plant, and is normally smoked.

Cocaine is a white powder that is snorted, sniffed, swallowed, smoked, and injected. The most common method is sniffing or snorting. Cocaine may be found packaged in baggies, vials, and similar containers. It is frequently laid out in "lines" on a smooth surface to be inhaled into the nose with a small tube or straw. Cocaine use may cause runny nose, paranoia, depression, irritability, violent behavior, headaches, and trouble sleeping.

Crack is a dangerous and deadly form of cocaine. It appears on the street as small white, brown, or tan pellets, rocks, or chips. It is inhaled through a pipe or similar device and is 5 to 10 times more potent than cocaine that is snorted through the nose. Crack provides a quick, intense, but short-lived "high", and then results in a need for more of the drug. Some of the effects of crack use are weight loss, hyperactivity, hoarseness and heart attack. Crack can addict the user faster than any other drug!

Inhalants such as gasoline, glue, spray paints, rubber cement, and other chemicals can cause a "high" when inhaled. They can also cause permanent damage to the nervous system, liver, kidneys, and can lead to various psychological problems.

Some athletes inject anabolic steroids in order to improve their physical ability and appearance. Steroid use can cause liver damage, testicle atrophy, aggressive behavior, high cholesterol, high risk for heart attack, enlarged prostate, baldness, depression, and other problems.

Possible signs of drug use are:

- Appears intoxicated or drunk
- Wears sunglasses to hide red eyes
- Starts using incense or other deodorizers
- The smell of Marijuana
  (some say it smells like burnt rope)
- Presence of drug paraphernalia
- Mood swings
- Failing or dropping grades in school
- Reports of skipping or dropping classes
- Missing complete days in school
- Pays less attention to responsibilities
- Always needing money
- Arrests or tickets for vehicle incidents
- Selling personal items
- Valuables missing from the home
- Spending more time away from home
- Wants more privacy

There are many things that could be considered signs of drug use and abuse. Some could indicate medical or other problems. Get all the facts. Consult a professional.

Chapter 2

Drugs and AIDS

Aids is a disease that attacks the body's immune system. As the disease progresses, the body becomes unable to fight off diseases such as cancer, pneumonia, and tuberculosis the way a healthy body can. The major avenues of infection with the AIDS virus are sharing needles used to inject drugs, intimate sexual relations and receiving AIDS contaminated blood, or allowing AIDS contaminated blood or body fluids to enter your bloodstream.

There have been no reported cases of the AIDS virus being transmitted by shaking hands, hugging, or from toilet seats.

However, using alcohol or other drugs can ruin your judgment about activities that lead to AIDS!

CHAPTER 3

Drugs and Gangs

The number of street gangs and the incidence of violence involving them is definitely on the rise. If you live in a large city, you know this already. If you live in a smaller or medium size city, you have probably seen stories about it on your local television, or are beginning to experience the problem locally.

One of the reasons gangs form is out of the feeling for a need to band together. This feeling is for protection against other groups with conflicting interests or intentions.

It is generally believed that gangs are made up of members of society who fit a certain mold. People who join gangs are usually "followers" who are not able to get respect without their "gang identity". There are many reasons why people join gangs and you would have to uncover the truth with facts.

They probably had no one in their lives to provide a positive influence on them. They were probably left home alone a lot due to various circumstances. They may have been involved in minor crimes and possibly drug use. They lack any feeling of importance or power. They have no real self-esteem. They feel there is no excitement in their lives.

Gang-related graffiti is one sure sign of the presence of or the impending emergence of gang activity in your area. Gangs mark their turf with gang symbols which can be found on building walls, fences, sidewalks, and on just about anything else in the neighborhood. These gang symbols and other markings can contain very complicated codes.

- Some gangs and/or members are very well armed.
- Change in attitude about society, authority, etc.
- Riding around in cars filled with people.
- School work suffering and class attendance dropping.
- Gang graffiti near or at your home.
- Use of alcohol or drugs.
- Being secretive about their activities.
- Wearing a different style of clothing and hanging out with others who dress the same.
- Strange or threatening phone calls, possibly from rival gang members, to your home.

Chapter 4

Advice for Youth on Drugs

Drugs do absolutely NOTHING for you! Those who use or sell drugs will end up with nothing but a sick, broken body, a police record, no real job, or DEAD! You can do better than that!

Graduating from high school can make it possible for you to earn several hundred thousand dollars MORE during your working life than someone who only finished the eighth grade or dropped out of high school.

Are you thinking of being a teacher, airline pilot, nurse, doctor, lawyer, psychologist, dentist, veterinarian, optometrist, or fighter pilot? Don't even think about dropping out. These are all college graduates.

Many jobs that only required a high school diploma a few years ago are now going to people with a college background. With so many people looking for work, employers can now pick from only the best.

Don't pick up hypodermic needles or syringes you see on the ground or in the trash. They can carry viruses that cause diseases including hepatitis and AIDS.

Check with your police agency about Law Enforcement Exploring. You'll have a great time and you'll learn a lot, too. If your agency doesn't have a post ask them to start one.

Some drugs can kill you the first time you try them!

Be very alert around strangers. The sad truth is that there are people in the world who will hurt you for no reason. Be aware of where you are and who is around you at all times.

Your mom and dad said it. Your teacher said it. Now here it is again: NEVER GET INTO A CAR WITH A STRANGER! You may never be seen again! Run away from anyone who tries to get you into a car. Scream, yell, and RUN!

You come home from school and find the door to your house open. No one is supposed to be at home. STOP right there and go to a responsible neighbor's house, the nearest pay phone, or other location designated by your parents, and call the police! Do not go into the house! Do not walk around the house to check other windows and doors! If you walk in on a burglar, you could be injured, kidnapped, or killed! Let the police check the house!

Never tell strangers, in person or over the phone, how many people are in your family, when your mom and dad go to work or come home, or anything else that will let someone know when it's a good time to break into your home.

Always wear a seat belt when traveling in a car. Many accidents can injure or kill you, and many will make you crack the windshield with your face and make you ugly for the rest of your life! Or paralyzed!

Don't let your friends talk you into doing something dangerous or against the law. Don't ruin your day or your life on a dare. Stop and think... then decide.

Don't play with guns! Don't hang around someone else who is playing with a gun. Get away as fast as you can and tell your parents! Bullets can travel over a mile, and through walls, and injure or kill you!

Don't use steroids! You don't need them. Steroids can't replace a hard workout! Don't drink. When you drink it's hard to make the right decisions.

Chapter 5

Drug Street Names

Street names for drugs change quite often, so it is important to stay abreast of common terms if you suspect a family member is using them. Below are the common slang terms for illegal drugs, and then we list a mini drug dictionary so you can become familiar with the meanings. Of course there are more drug terms and names, but we are just giving you the most popular terms and names. If you suspect someone is using illegal drugs, then help them to an addiction or drug rehabilitation center. There are many centers throughout the nation, and you can get more information from your local law enforcement agency.

Street Names and Slang for Hallucinogens

Marijuana
- Pot
- Reefer
- Grass
- Weed
- Dope
- Ganja
- Mary Jane
- Sinsemilla
- Urb
- 420
- Aunt Mary
- Baby

- Bobby
- Boom
- Chira
- Chronic
- Ditch greens
- Hash
- Herb
- Nigra
- Rip
- Root
- Skunk
- Stack
- Torch
- Zambi
- Loud

Hashish

- Hash

Mescaline and Peyote

- Mesc
- Buttons
- Cactus
- Beans
- Cactus buttons
- Cactus head
- Chief
- Love trip
- Mesc
- Mescal
- Mezc
- Moon
- Peyote
- Topi.

Psilocybin (Shrooms)

- Magic Mushrooms
- 'shrooms
- Boomers
- God's flesh
- Little smoke
- Mexican mushrooms
- Mushrooms
- Musk
- Sherm
- Silly putty
- Simple simon.

Lysergic acid diethylamide

- Acid
- Microdot
- White lightning
- Blue heaven
- Sugar Cubes
- A
- Black star
- Blotter
- Boomers
- Cubes
- Elvis
- Golden dragon
- L
- Paper acid
- Pink robots
- Superman
- Twenty-five
- Yellow sunshine
- Ying yang

Analog of Amphetamines or Methamphetamines

- MDMA (Ecstasy, XTC, Adam, Essence)
- MDM
- STP
- PMA
- 2
- 5-DMA
- TMA
- DOM
- DOB
- EVE

Phencyclidine

- PCP
- Hog
- Angel Dust
- Loveboat
- Lovely

Analog of Phencyclidine (PCP)

- PCPy
- PCE
- Angel dust
- Belladonna
- Black whack
- CJ
- Cliffhanger
- Crystal joint
- Detroit pink
- Elephant tranquilizer
- Hog
- Magic
- Peter Pan
- Sheets

- Soma
- TAC
- Trank
- White horizon
- Zoom

Street Names and Slang for Depressants

Nitrous Oxide
- Laughing gas
- Whippets

Amyl Nitrite
- Poppers
- Snappers

Butyl Nitrite
- Rush
- Bolt
- Bullet
- Locker Room
- Climax

Chlorohydrocarbons
- Aerosol sprays
- Cleaning fluids

Hydrocarbons
- Solvents

Barbiturates
- Downers
- Barbs

- Blue Devils
- Red Devils
- Yellow Jackets
- Yellows
- Nembutal
- Tuinals
- Seconal
- Amytal

Methaqualone

- Quaaludes
- Ludes
- Sopors

Rohypnol/Flunitrazepam

- Circles
- Forget-me pill
- La rocha
- Lunch money drug
- Mexican valium
- Pingus
- Reynolds
- Roche
- Roofies
- Rope
- Ruffles
- Wolfies

- Date rape drug
- La roche
- R2
- Rib
- Roach
- Roofenol
- Roofies
- Rope
- Rophies
- Ruffies
- The forget pill

Tranquilizers
- Valium
- Librium
- Serax
- Equanil
- Miltown
- Tranxene

Street Names and Slang for Stimulants

Cocaine
- Coke
- Snow
- Nose Candy
- Flake
- Blow

- Big C
- Lady
- White
- Snowbirds
- Powder
- C
- Candy
- Do a line
- Freeze
- Girl
- Happy dust
- Mama coca
- Mojo
- Monster
- Nose
- Pimp
- Shot
- Smoking gun sugar
- Sweet stuff
- White powder

Crack Cocaine

- Crack
- Rock
- Freebase
- Cookie
- Base
- Beat
- Blast
- Casper
- Chalk
- Devil drug
- Gravel
- Hardball

- Hell
- Kryptonite
- Love
- Moonrocks
- Rock
- Scrabble
- Stones
- Tornado

Amphetamines

- Speed
- Uppers
- Ups
- Black beauties
- Pep pills
- Co-pilots
- Bumblebees
- Hearts
- Benzedrine
- Dexedrine
- Footballs
- Biphetamine

Methamphetamines

- Crank
- Crystal meth
- Crystal methadrine
- Speed
- Beannies
- Blue devils
- Chalk
- CR
- Crystal
- Fast

- Granulated orange
- Ice
- Meth
- Mexican crack
- Pink
- Rock
- Speckled birds
- Tina
- Yellow powder

Methcathinone

- Bathtub speed
- Cadillac express
- Cat
- Crank
- Ephedrone
- Gagers
- Go-fast
- Goob
- Qat
- Slick superspeed
- Star
- The C
- Tweeker
- Wild cat
- Wonder star

Additional Stimulants

- Ritalin (Crackers, One and ones, Pharming, Poor man's heroin, R-ball, Ritz an ts, Set, Skippy, Speedball, Ts and ritz, Ts and rs, Vitamin R, and West coast.
- Cylert
- Preludin
- Didrex
- Pre-State
- Voranil
- Sandrex
- Plegine

Street Names and Slang for Narcotics

Heroin

- Smack
- Horse
- Mud
- Brown sugar
- Junk
- Black tar
- Big H
- Aunt Hazel
- Black pearl
- Capital H
- Charley
- China white
- Dope
- Good horse
- H
- Hard stuff

- Hero
- Heroina
- Little boy
- Perfect high
- Stuff
- Tar

Morphine

- Pectoral syrup

Opium

- Paregoric
- Dover's Powder
- Parepectolin
- Ah-pen-yen
- Aunti
- Big O
- Black stuff
- Chinese tobacco
- Chocolate
- Dopium
- Dover's deck
- Dream gun
- Hard stuff
- Hocus
- Joy plant
- O
- Ope
- Pin yen
- Toxy
- Zero

Codeine

- Empirin compound with codeine
- Tylenol with codeine
- Codeine in cough medicine

Meperidine

- Pethidine
- Demerol
- Mepergan

Analog of Fentanyl (Narcotic)

- Synthetic heroin
- China white
- Apache
- China girl
- China town
- Dance fever
- Friend
- Goodfellas
- Great bear
- He-man
- Jackpot
- King ivory
- Murder 8
- Poison
- Tango and cash
- TNT.

Analog of Meperidine (Narcotic)

- MPTP (New heroin)
- MPPP
- Synthetic heroin

Addictive

The property of a drug that can cause a psychological or physical dependence.

AIDS

Acquired Immune Deficiency Syndrome. A fatal disease that attacks and destroys the body's immune system. This disease makes the body unable to fight off infections and other disease. As the condition progresses and the body becomes weaker, diseases such as cancer, tuberculosis and pneumonia take hold and cause the death of the victim. AIDS is found frequently in people who have shared needles with other people while injecting intravenous drugs.

Angel Dust

Another name for the hallucinogen PCP.

Atom Bomb

A name for the mixture of heroin and marijuana.

Barbiturates

A class of depressants often prescribed by doctors to help people sleep. Barbiturates are taken orally and are sold on the illegal drug market. Phenobarbital is a widely known barbiturate.

Clandestine (clandestine laboratories)

Describes secret, or hidden, laboratories where illegal drugs are manufactured.

Cocaine
Made from the leaf of the coca plant that is grown in South America. It stimulates the nervous system and has mind-altering effects. Cocaine can constrict the blood vessels which causes the heart to strain in order to do its work. Repeated cocaine use can cause a psychological dependence that becomes the most important thing in the user's life. Cocaine use during pregnancy can cause miscarriages and even stillbirth.

Colors
The colored insignia, flags, bandanas, or other items that indicate specific gang or club affiliation.

Crack
A very dangerous form of cocaine that is sometimes called "rock" because it resembles small rock or stone chips, rock salt, soap chips or crystals. It is white or tan in color. It is normally smoked. Crack use can cause a very high heart rate and possible heart attack. This can happen even with the first use! It causes a very strong "high" and then a very devastating "crash"!

Crank
A name given to the mixture of cocaine and heroin that is usually injected. Since the arrival of crack, this name also applies to the mixture of crack and the smokable form of heroin. These mixtures are also known as "speedball".

Depressants
Drugs that cause a relaxing, intoxicating effect. Often called tranquilizers. Some common types are Tuinal, Seconal, Miltown, Librium, Valium, and Chloral Hydrate.

DWI

Driving while intoxicated. This is the charge filed against a person arrested for drunk driving. In many states a driver is presumed to be intoxicated to a degree where he is a danger to himself or others when his blood alcohol level is 0.10% or more. Some states call the offense DUI, or "driving under the influence". Some states have a separate charge for driving under the influence of drugs, or DUID. Some states make no distinction.

Dusted
Under the influence of PCP.

Dusting
Adding PCP or other drugs to marijuana.

Ecstasy
The most popular of the "designer drugs". It is sometimes taken as an aphrodisiac, but its effects can be the opposite of what the user intended or expected. This drug can cause blurred vision, blood pressure changes, and even brain damage.

Euphoria
A feeling of well-being. In this presentation it is used to describe an effect of a particular drug.

Freebasing
A term used to describe the smoking of cocaine after its active ingredient has been separated from its salt base. It is usually smoked in water-filled pipes. Heat applied to the bowl causes the "freebase" to vaporize. There is a risk of fire during this process due to the dangerous chemicals that must be used.

Goofball
A term for the mixture of cocaine and heroin.

Hallucination
An imagined seeing of visions or hearing of sounds.

Hallucinogens PCP LSD
As the name implies, hallucinogens cause the user to experience hallucinations. All the person's senses may become distorted and totally unreliable and unpredictable. They may lose all sense of reality.

Hashish
A dark brown, but sometimes green or black, resin that is derived from the marijuana plant. Hashish is smoked in pipes or similar devices. Hashish oil is usually smoked by putting it on regular cigarettes or marijuana cigarettes.

Herb and Al
A name for marijuana and alcohol.

Hyperactivity
Abnormally high level of activity.

Hypodermic Needle/Syringe
The syringe is a hollow barrel containing a plunger inside. It is tipped with a hollow needle. It is used to inject drugs under the skin. Hypodermic means "under the skin".

Ice
A very dangerous, crystallized form of methamphetamine. It is believed that ICE originated in Hawaii. It looks like rock candy or rock salt. ICE is made into its solid or crystallized form by cooking it. ICE can be even more dangerous and

addictive than cocaine or crack. ICE is virtually odorless when smoked.

Illicit (illicit drug use - illicit drugs)
Used in this presentation to describe the illegal use of prescription drugs or the use of illegal drugs.

Inhalants
Chemicals that are introduced into the body by breathing or inhaling them. Common inhalants are spray paints, glue, felt markers, polishes, and gasoline. These are legal, easily obtained items, but contains poisons that cause a "high" when purposely inhaled in concentrated amounts. Spray paints (gold and silver are popular) are sprayed into paper or plastic sacks. The sack is then placed over the mouth and nose and the concentrated fumes inhaled. The chemicals can also be poured or sprayed onto rags and held against the face. The effects range from lightheadedness to intoxication to coma. "Sniffing" ("huffing") causes brain damage (usually irreversible)! It also damages other vital organs such as the liver, kidneys, and lungs.

Intoxication
Being under the influence of alcohol, drugs, or other chemical. Being drunk.

Intravenous
Injected or introduced directly into the vein.

Junkie
A person who is addicted to drugs.

Mescaline
A white, crystalline substance derived from the tops of a species of cactus. It can cause hallucinations.

Methamphetamines
The most popular stimulant. Sometimes called "speed", "uppers", "crank", or "crystal". Methamphetamines are taken due to their effect of causing increased alertness and euphoria. An overdose can cause a stroke or heart attack.

Nicotine
A very poisonous chemical found in tobacco.

Opium
A poisonous and addictive chemical derived from the poppy plant.
Morphine and codeine are derived from it.

Paraphernalia (drug)
Equipment or apparatus used to assist in the smoking or injection of drugs. Syringes, needles, roach clips, spoons, etc.

Paranoia
A mental condition describing a feeling of persecution. This condition is brought on by the use of certain drugs.

PCP (Phencyclidine)
Considered to be the most dangerous of the hallucinogens. PCP has many different street names including, angel dust and supergrass. PCP was first produced as an anesthetic, but is now made only in clandestine labs.

Roach Clip

Any device used to hold the short butt (roach) of a marijuana cigarette. Small "alligator" clips are very common.

Speed

See "Methamphetamine".

Speedball

A term used for the mixture of cocaine and heroin. Since the arrival of crack, the term now more frequently applies to the mixture of crack and heroin in its smokable form.

Steroids

Hormones used to enhance physical ability, strength, and appearance of the user. It is generally thought that the hazards associated with steroid use far outweigh any possible benefit. It is often considered a drug because of its effects, but it is a hormone.

Stimulants

A class of drugs that causes an increase in energy, alertness, and possibly activity. Some examples are Benzedrine, Preludin, Fastin, Ritalin and amphetamines. Continued use of stimulants can cause weight loss, mood changes, tremors, and palpitations.

Tragic Magic

A term for the mixture of PCP and crack.

Zoom

A mixture of PCP and marijuana.

Afterword

If you have a friend who is using drugs of any type, talk to him or her and let them know you care about what may happen to their life because of their actions. Don't just point your finger at them and talk down to them. Really show them you care and are willing to help them get the help they need. But remember not to let yourself be caught in suspicious places or circumstances with someone who may have drugs on them. It is possible that you could be arrested, depending on the situation, if you are with someone who is caught with drugs!

If your friend does not listen to you, ask your parents for advice on how to handle the situation. Your parents can be your best source of guidance if you give them a chance.

Your friend may need medical attention or counseling for the problem. You can also get information and advice from your school, religious, holistic consultants, or professional substance abuse counselors. A good detox is needed for at least 2-4 weeks to help restore the body back to balance. Also, a good holistic consultation would reveal the cause of the drug abuse. After all, the usage of drugs is only an effect of the real cause.

We hope this guide has been informative and helpful for you. It can be a reference guide for years as an educational source on preventing the use of illegal drugs.

About the Author

Franklin Gillette

Franklin Gillette was born on July 7, 1971 in Chicago, Illinois. Through the years, he has grown to uncover his gifts and purpose as a Visionary, Humanitarian, Motivational speaker, Author, Natural Health Consultant, Entrepreneur.

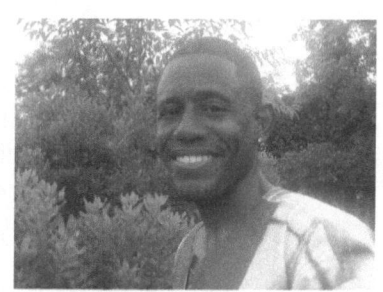

Franklin Gillette, originator of the *Automatic Natural Weight Loss System*, also specializes in helping people restore good health by aligning with the body's natural systems and cycles. Moreover, his best-selling book, *Compatibility: Code of Harmony for Love and Unity*, reflects his expertise in relationships as an expression of oneness.

Franklin Gillette provides consultations, coaching, seminars, workshops, and books on all levels for happiness and success. He presently resides in Maryland with his beautiful wife Sereda.

Find Franklin Gillette on Facebook, Twitter, YouTube, LinkedIn, Lulu, Goodreads, and Google+.

You may reach Franklin Gillette at:
allowoneness@gmail.com

One Last Thing

I appreciate you reading this wonderful book of mine. The highest thanks you can give me is leaving a review on the site or venue you bought this from (Lulu, iBookstore, Nook, etc.), and also referring my book(s) to family and friends.

Thank you!

Franklin Gillette
allowoneness@gmail.com

Compatibility has been known by many to mean many things. It has widely been associated with astrology, which helps to determine if one person can get along with the other person. When you are finished reading this book, you will see that compatibility is much more than that. There is a certain code, like a combination lock, that will unlock the tools necessary to apply and establish mutual love and unity once again. This book is universal and is beneficial for the

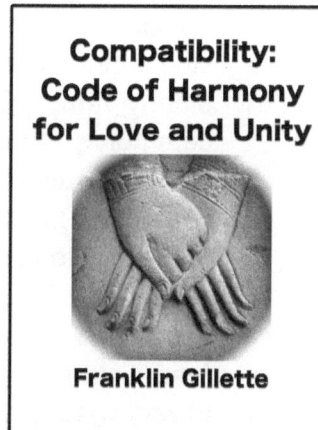

Compatibility: Code of Harmony for Love and Unity

Franklin Gillette

individual, couple, group, or society. The code to compatibility has been scattered throughout the world like pieces to a puzzle. This book, Compatibility The Code of Harmony For Love & Unity, will give you the knowledge necessary to put the pieces of the puzzle back together. You will find that this book is the ultimate guide for solving any type of relationship issue once and for all. There isn't a book, guide, or manual that covers more information on compatibility than this book, Compatibility The Code of Harmony For Love & Unity.

Price $4.99 (ePub), $14.99 (paperback)
ISBN 9781105908187
Copyright Franklin Gillette
(Creative Commons Attribution 2.0)
Edition Second Edition
Published December 21, 2013
Pages 231
File Format ePub
File Size 164.31 KB

Visit here for this title and more!
http://bit.ly/JmVJ5E

This book is for the individual, single mother, student, disabled, elderly, family, group, and community. If you want to ensure a safe environment for yourself or family, then this book has the potential of possibly saving your life! It is not meant to live and walk around in a fearful state of mind. However, it is very wise to do all you practically can to build a strong

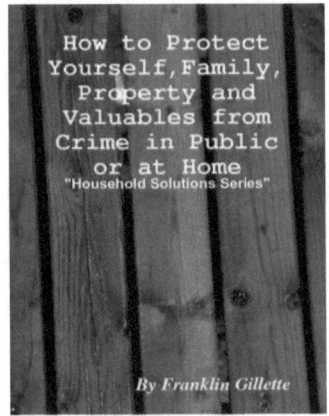

defense and fortress for protection. Even if you are confident in your security measures, you can this book to someone you love who may not be as prepared. You cannot be everywhere at all times, so it helps to have everyone on the same page to ensure a safe environment mentally and physically.

Unless you live in a bubble, this book is a necessary book that you should have and implement into your daily lives. Each chapter focuses on an action that could ease your mind of losing someone or something dear to you.

eBook $1.99
Paperback $6.99
ISBN 9781304791832
Edition First Edition
Publisher Lulu Press
Published January 9, 2014
Pages 75
Binding Perfect-bound Paperback
Dimensions (inches) 6 wide x 9 tall
http://www.lulu.com/spotlight/FranklinGillette

www.ingramcontent.com/pod-product-compliance
Lightning Source LLC
Chambersburg PA
CBHW030105300526
45785CB00019B/2729